WHAT OTHERS ARE SAYING ABOUT

"The need for a book like this ... dementia and strategies fami... dealing with it in clear, unders...uable language, with plenty of concrete examples. Thank you, Memory Care!"

—**Lewis C. Chartock, PhD**

"Excellent information for caregivers in a simple, clear manner that is uncluttered with jargon makes these tips easy to apply to one's daily life."

—**Marylen Mann**
Chairman of the Board of OASIS

"The clearly written narratives, success stories and tips found in this book not only gives the reader hope in caring for a loved one who has Alzheimer's disease, but also expresses how to preserve the dignity of the person."

—**Brother Warren Longo, CFA**
Assistant Superior General
Congregation of Alexian Brothers

"This comprehensive guide explains symptoms and solutions and offers helpful, practical information for caregivers."

—**Brian Carpenter, PhD**
Associate Professor Dept. of Psychology
Washington University in St. Louis

"This book is wonderful! It offers a variety of insightful information for caregivers about what to expect from their loved ones as they progress through their dementia and provides easy steps to take in order to handle their deteriorating memories and keep them safely at home longer."

—Barth Holohan, MSW, MBA
President of Continuum Care and Family Partners
Adult Day Services

Memory Care Guidebook

Memory Care Guidebook

Strategies and solutions for family caregivers

**Prepared by Harriet Rzetelny, LCSW
in conjunction with
Memory Care Home Solutions**

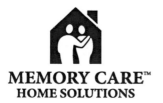

MEMORY CARE™
HOME SOLUTIONS

ISBN: 978-0-615-41130-9
Library of Congress Control Number: 2010942167

Book designed by Nehmen-Kodner: www.n-kcreative.com
Printed in the United States of America

Published by Memory Care Home Solutions
www.memorycarehs.org • help@memorycarehs.org
1526 South Big Bend Boulevard, St. Louis, MO 63117
314-645-6247

THIS BOOK IS DEDICATED TO THE MILLIONS OF FAMILIES, FRIENDS, and professional caregivers who tirelessly give of themselves to create the best life possible for those at home experiencing memory loss and dementia. We hope the information in this book will ease some of their burdens by providing concrete solutions to the everyday problems that arise out of living with and caring for such a person, be they spouse, parent, sister, brother, friend, significant other, or patient.

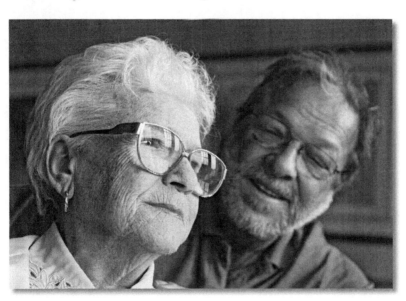

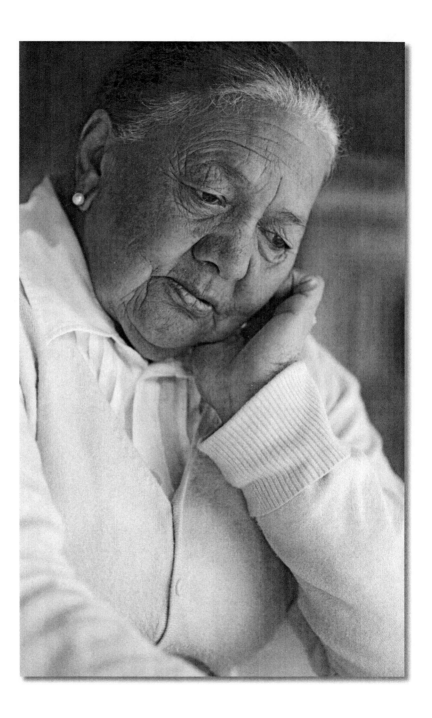

Contents

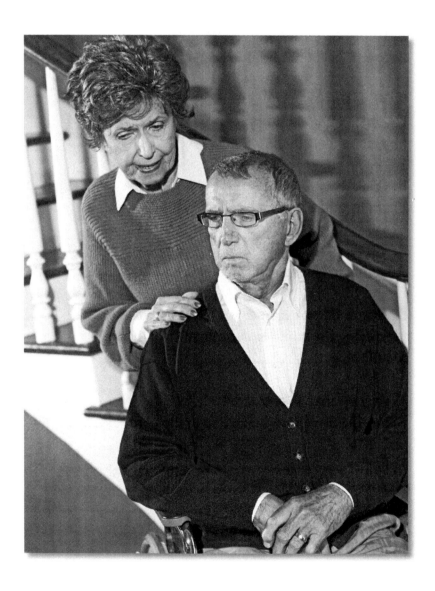

Acknowledgments

This guidebook exists primarily due to the generous funding received from the Mildred, Herbert and Julian Simon Foundation. We are especially grateful to Harriet Rzetelny, LCSW, who authored both the Memory Care In-Home Training Curriculum and this guidebook. Her sensitivity and keen insight into caregivers made the training curriculum and this guidebook the unique and helpful tools that they are. Geriatric care specialist Stefanie Osiek, MA, assisted Ms. Rzetelny by providing practical solutions and caregiving examples from loving and dedicated families. Some caregiver stories are composites, but all illustrate real problems and the strategies caregivers adopted to deal with them. Steve Miskovic, MSW, spearheaded the administrative and content oversight that led to the guidebook's finalization and printing.

The Board of Directors of Memory Care Home Solutions, volunteer Guidebook Chair Pat Chartock, PhD, and the Barnes-Jewish Hospital In-Home Services Department gave valuable input to the organization and the content of this guidebook.

The Program Director came to our home in January and was very patient, understanding and sympathetic to our needs. He was very thorough in explaining the different stages of dementia and what we could expect in the weeks, months and years to come. We received excellent suggestions and recommendations on handling transitions in our day-to-day living.

— Lois

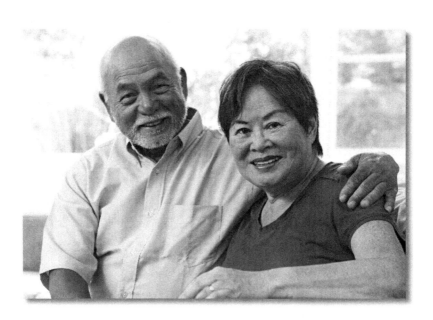

Introduction

IF YOU ARE LOOKING FOR A BASIC BOOK ON ALZHEIMER'S disease, this is not the book for you. This book begins where those books leave off: with the how-to's of everyday, at-home caregiving.

Of the five million Americans experiencing dementia, 75 percent are being cared for at home. It is clear that families want to keep their loved ones at home for as long as possible, but need concrete, practical help in order to do so.

If you are a family member about to read this book, you probably have no training in what to do when the person you are caring for:

- simply refuses to wash herself or brush her teeth
- screams, yells, and throws things
- paces around the room endlessly
- accuses you or other family members of being a thief
- rummages through closets and drawers
- wanders away from home

Caring for a person with dementia who is living at home takes patience, planning, and know-how—but it can be done! How do we know? Many families very much like yours are doing it. This book contains strategies and solutions for common problems that are based on the experiences of the many families and health care professionals who have already "walked the road." The guidebook includes many caregiver stories that illustrate how different families handled particular problems. Not all of their strategies and solutions will work for everyone, nor is there one right answer to every problem. Try some of the ones we suggest, or create ones of your own. If a solution works, it's the right one for you.

You will hear this and we can't stress it enough: You can't do it alone. Besides the emotional price, family caregivers experience a huge financial toll, with average lifetime out-of-pocket cost of $175,000 per family, as of this writing (2010). So the guidebook includes a resource section with additional information about dementia, caregiving assistance, and other services to help ease your burden. You'll be amazed by how much help is available, including the services and programs of Memory Care Home Solutions. If you don't already know about Memory Care Home Solutions, visit our website at **www.memorycarehs.org.**

A note to health care professionals on the use of this guidebook: The majority of family caregivers who use Memory Care Home Solutions services are either elderly spouses or adult children struggling to provide care in the home with limited resources and how-to knowledge. The guidebook targets the most common problems family caregivers face in their daily lives, and offers simple, inexpensive solutions that can easily be adapted to their home situations.

Whether you are a family caregiver or a professional health care provider, this guidebook will be a valuable tool because it shares solutions from families facing the same daily challenges of caring for someone with dementia at home.

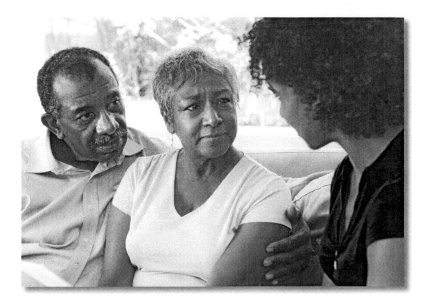

To Lisa:

I want to take this opportunity to tell you how helpful the Memory Care Home Solutions social worker has been in times that we all know are challenging. In dealing with my husband's illness, I've been blessed with incredible support from family and friends. I could not continue, however, without the contributions the social worker made, the ongoing excellence of the care at the adult day program, and the medical advice of our outstanding neurologist. The social worker helped me accept the place that day services could have in keeping home-based care doable. It was a very hard decision and his input was invaluable. I don't know anyone else dealing with our problems, but I would certainly suggest Memory Care Home Solutions should I find out someone is dealing with Alzheimer's disease or related disorders. It is an important community resource.

Thank you,
— Sheila

1

Home Is Where the Heart Is
An overview of home-based caregiving

Who is a caregiver?

Caregivers come from every walk of life. Caregivers can be men or women (although most of us are female), rich or poor, or any place in between, and can come from any ethnic, racial, or cultural group. We can be spouses, children, sisters or brothers, or loving friends. For many of us, caregiving is a natural and expected part of our adult experience. In the course of our lives we may care for one or both parents, in-laws, sisters or brothers, husbands, or wives. We may live jointly with the person we care for, we may live close by, or we may live hundreds or thousands of miles away. We may be sole caregivers, or we may have other family members with whom we share responsibilities. We may be single or live with our own families. Or we may function as paid caregivers to people who are not family members. If you are reading this guidebook, you are probably already a caregiver or about to become one.

The rewards of caregiving

Although this guidebook focuses on finding solutions to *problems* that confront you as caregivers, it is important to look at some of the *rewards* that you may also experience as caregivers. Here are some that have been reported to us:

- **Caring for those we love.** Many of us truly and deeply love the person we care for. Their happiness and well-being are important to us, and we want to help give them the best lives possible.

- **Giving back.** If the person you care for cared for you when you were a child, or during a sickness or disability, then providing care when the need arises is an opportunity to give back.

- **Doing the right thing.** Many of us have ethical, religious, or moral beliefs that tell us to "do unto others as you would have them do unto you." Some believe that caring for others in need is the highest form of love. Whatever your reasons, caregiving may feel "right" to you.

- **A sense of satisfaction.** Providing care to someone in a way that helps them maintain a good quality of life, especially when it involves using problem-solving abilities, can feel like "a job well done" and bring us a sense of satisfaction.

A word about strategies and solutions

How do you begin to solve those everyday problems that arise when you are caring for someone with dementia? We first try to find solutions. For example, if your wife cannot get out of the bathtub unassisted, a solution might be to install a handrail next to the tub. In another case, if your out-of-state sister plans to care for your mother while you take a well-earned vacation, but your sister hasn't taken care of Mom before, a solution could be to write out a detailed schedule of your mother's daily activities, including likes and dislikes, and post it on the refrigerator.

Other problems, such as your father's agitated pacing around the house, frequent upsets, and other kinds of disturbing behavior may appear resistant to easy solutions, as indeed they are. They require a deeper understanding of what might be causing the problem, and a longer-term strategy to help you to deal with it. Although it is outside the scope of this guidebook to explain the physiological changes in the brain that cause dementia, we will help you understand the kinds of everyday problems that arise from these changes, as well as provide strategies and solutions to help you deal with them.

The terms **strategies** and **solutions** are often used interchangeably, but they actually mean two different things. A **strategy** is the overall plan or approach to a set of problems that is based on understanding the cause, or causes, of the problem. A **solution** is an immediate answer to a particular problem and arises from the strategy or approach you choose. In other words, strategies are guidelines for helping you find solutions.

This guidebook presents stories about common problems that family caregivers face. Each story discusses how family caregivers use an overall strategy that helps guide them to find solutions.

▪ Strategies & Solutions ▪

Connie was a widow who lived with her mother, Mrs. T., who had Alzheimer's disease. Mrs. T. got very agitated and upset at the least little thing: when the doorbell rang, when she was not able to find an item of clothing, or when she did not understand something Connie said. When Mrs. T. got agitated, she yelled, stomped around, and waved her hands wildly. She even hit Connie a few times. Connie knew she needed to think of ways of reducing her mother's agitation. The first strategy that Connie used was to give her mother medication to reduce her agitation. But Mrs. T.'s doctor could not find a suitable medication that Mrs. T. could tolerate in a dosage high enough to reduce her agitation without producing unwanted side effects.

As a second strategy, Connie tried changing her own behavior and their home setting to reduce Mrs. T.'s agitation. Connie attended a workshop on family caregiving and decided to try some of the techniques she learned. Here are two solutions she tried and found successful:

1) By using simple sentences, Connie was able to help her mother understand what she was trying to say.

2) By putting pictures on her mother's closet and dresser, Connie helped Mrs. T. identify the contents and Mrs. T. was able to find the clothing she wanted.

Both of these solutions helped lessen Mrs. T.'s agitation.

———————

The three factors that contribute to problems in the home

If you look closely at most caregiving problems that occur at home, you will usually find that there are three factors at work:

1. The person with dementia
2. You, the caregiver, and your family
3. Your home environment

Let's look at each of these factors.

1. The person with dementia

All people with dementia have some kind of memory loss and confusion, problems with understanding and using complex language, irrational outbursts, and behaviors that may seem purposeless or unexplainable, but that does not mean that they are all alike. (See Chapter 2 for a further description of these and other problems associated with dementia.) Nor does dementia cause the person who has it to suddenly become someone else, although it may seem that way at times.

People's basic personalities, their likes and dislikes, remain fairly stable throughout life. If your mother liked to cook and play cards before she developed dementia, she will probably continue to enjoy doing these activities, although she may not be able to cook an entire meal or play a hand of canasta. If your husband liked woodworking, he will probably still enjoy working with wood although he may not be able to build a bookcase or repair a broken chair. If your father was always a loner, he will most likely continue to enjoy more solitary activities after he develops dementia. Some of the behavioral changes that you see are a reaction to the disease as the person with dementia becomes frightened, anxious, or depressed over what is happening to him. Other changes arise from the disease as dementia robs him of his ability to control his speech, actions, or behaviors. Later sections of the guidebook explain ways all family caregivers can involve their loved one in traditional family activities that he or she previously enjoyed, but in more simplified ways.

People with dementia cannot adapt to your needs because of the disease affecting their brain. You must adapt to theirs.

In order to adapt to somcone's needs, you must first identify those needs and then be able to change your own behavior in response to the individual's. People with dementia lose awareness of what other people are thinking and feeling, and they cannot change or control their behavior in any kind of purposeful way. You can learn to manage their behaviors (see Chapter 6 on Managing Difficult Behaviors), but any solutions you select mean adapting to their needs. For example, if you need quiet in order to do some paperwork in the living room, you can't expect your mother to remain quiet simply because you ask her to. You must come up with a strategy that involves either doing your paperwork after she goes to sleep or finding a quiet activity for her like watching TV or listening to soft music.

■ Strategies & Solutions ■

Bill was a caregiver to his wife, Jean. When he and Jean were driving together in the car, Jean fooled around with the knobs and buttons on the dashboard. This was very distracting for Bill and potentially created a dangerous situation. He told her to stop doing it, but she still continued. Jean's inability to grasp the dangerous situation was due to her disease. Once he realized that she did not understand the dangers her behavior created, he knew he'd have to change how he handled her behavior. His first solution was to have her sit in the backseat and lock the door. But this got her very upset and she banged on his head and tried to reach over the seat.

Next, he tried distracting her. She had always enjoyed making scrapbooks and other craft activities. He bought a set of small magnetized objects—such as colorful insects, flowers, and animals—and a magnetic board for her to use. He put all these objects into a clear box and gave it to her when they drove. While they drove, she happily arranged and rearranged the objects and no longer touched the dashboard.

Craft stores are great places to find simple activities to distract and occupy people with dementia who enjoy doing things with their hands.

"She could do better if she wanted to." The truth is, she probably can't.

Sometimes caregivers believe that the person with dementia could "do a little more if they just tried a little harder." It is painfully hard to watch your mother, your father, your spouse deteriorating little by little. Just because your mother was able to button her coat last month by herself doesn't mean she can do it today. Like the rest of us, people with dementia have bad days and good days. Try to accept that your mother is probably doing the best she can at the moment. You can remind her to button her coat, but if that doesn't work, simply guide her hands to the buttons, or do it for her.

Ask yourself what could be causing the problem.

People with dementia typically cannot tell you what is bothering or upsetting them. They will often act out behaviorally instead. Try to treat situations like puzzles. Is he hot or cold? Is it too loud or noisy in the room? Are her allergies bothering her? Is he trying to do something that is now too hard for him? If you can't figure it out, ask someone who has experience in this area, such as homecare social workers, workshop leaders, and other caregivers, for tips and suggestions.

■ Strategies & Solutions ■

Lenny was the caregiver to his wife, Sally. Sally could no longer get the TV remote to work. As a result, she got upset and threw it across the room. At first, Lenny tried to help her by reminding her what the various buttons were used for. Unfortunately, his attempts upset her more and she continued to throw the remote across the room.

Lenny discussed the situation with the director of Sally's respite program. The director explained that Sally had lost her ability to understand what he had just told her about the remote buttons. Lenny's explanation of the remote, her inability to understand and remember, and her anxiety all caused Sally to feel overwhelmed and become even more upset. When he was able to understand the cause of the problem, he was able to solve it by the use of distraction. When Lenny saw that Sally was having trouble with the remote, he would call her into the kitchen for a snack. While she ate, he went into the den and put her favorite show on. After the snack, she returned to the den and was able to happily watch her program.

Remember the word 'distraction.' It often works when nothing else will.

---

2. The caregiver and the family

Just as no two people with dementia are alike, each caregiver and caregiving family is unique. People have different religious and moral beliefs and values; they come to caregiving with different life experiences, different personalities, and different levels of tolerance and understanding for certain kinds of behaviors. Because of these differences, a solution to a caregiving problem that will work for another family may not be the one that will work for you.

Know your own needs, tolerances, limitations, and strengths, and accept that those of your family members may be different than yours.

Some caregivers have a higher tolerance for disorder, for example, and won't get as upset if things are misplaced or not put away. Other caregivers are less tolerant of disorder and cannot function in surroundings that are not neat and orderly. Individual family members also differ from each other in their ability to understand and interact with the person who has dementia. Sometimes you, the primary caregiver, can accept and understand your mother's outbursts and odd behaviors, but your sister cannot and gets very upset. Or, conversely, your daughter may be able to talk to your father in a way that helps him to understand what she wants him to do in a way that you can't. The strategies and solutions you choose must take these differences within a caregiving family into account. Use the strengths that each family member possesses, and try to negotiate the differences.

Just a reminder (as if you didn't know): Caregiving is stressful!

Providing care at home to a person with dementia is one of life's most stressful undertakings. As the dementia progresses, and you have to take over more and more of the responsibility for the person you are caring for, your stress level will increase. You must first take care of yourself, or you cannot provide care to anyone else. Give yourself permission to take time away. Find someone to talk to. Join a support group. Learn relaxation techniques. Share the care with others in your family, if possible. Don't be a perfectionist—someone else may not know your relative as well, or provide the same quality of care as you do, but you can't do it alone. *Stress leads to less!* The more stressed you are, the less efficient, tolerant, adaptable, and good-humored you become, and the more vulnerable you are to stress-related diseases. (See Resources, page 115 for Caregiver

Support Groups and other resources to help you cope with stress.) Here are a few tips that our family caregivers have found particularly helpful:

Pick your battles. If you try to solve every problem that comes up, you will wear yourself out and probably be unsuccessful to boot. Focus on those problems that are really important to you and your family, and work on solving those.

Identify what you can and cannot change. If a problem arises from the disease condition, you probably can't change it. But you can change how you react to it. If your wife or mother cannot remember the name of something or someone no matter how many times you tell her, she will never remember it. If you find yourself getting really annoyed, maybe it's time to take a break yourself. Put on some music, find her something simple to do to distract her for a little while, and do something that you enjoy while she is doing it.

Don't sweat the small stuff. If your husband refuses to shave for a day or two no matter how much you try to help him, let him go unshaven. Eventually, the beard will begin to bother him, or he may be in a better mood, and you can try again.

Don't feel guilty because you are not the "perfect" caregiver. There is no such thing. You are doing the best you can. And, most important:

Try to keep your sense of humor!

3. The home environment

The term *home environment* means both the basic design of your house itself—such as the presence or absence of stairs, number of rooms, type of flooring, layout and other structural components—and the *general environment* within it—such as noise level, lighting arrangements, and the amount of clutter. It is necessary to adapt your home environment to the needs of the person with dementia in order to ensure his safety and security and help him remain as functional as possible. But each of you will develop an individualized plan on how to do this that is based on such issues as the basic design of your home, your family budget, your own needs and the needs of other family members, and the particular limitations and capacities of the person you are caring for. (See Chapter 5 on Home Modifications for more information about this topic.)

Home environment modifications need not be expensive.

Although some caregivers may elect to make extensive modifications such as adding an extra room, home modifications can involve as little as purchasing a shower seat, labeling closed cupboards to reflect their contents, and reducing noise and clutter. (See Chapter 5 for home modification suggestions and page 115 for resources.)

How do you select a strategy to guide you in problem-solving? Once you understand why a problem is occurring, the strategy you consider must be based on your and your family's needs, values, resources, and lifestyle.

Remember: There is no one strategy or solution that is right for everyone.

While many caregivers experience common problems such as caregiver stress, communication difficulties, and family discord, families will handle these problems in different ways.

▪ Strategies & Solutions ▪

Mary was a single mom raising two children, Lori, age 14, and Beth, age 16. Mary's mom, Mrs. R., had Alzheimer's disease and lived with them in their small apartment. Mary had an in-home training by a Memory Care Home

Solutions social worker, Steve, and learned that people with the disease retain their functional abilities longer if they're allowed to participate in activities with the family. Mary tried to follow this advice by encouraging her mother and daughters to eat dinner together. But mealtime became a nightmare. Lori and Beth were typical teenagers. During dinner, they talked and bickered in loud voices and their phones rang constantly. All of the noise and distraction agitated Mrs. R., who reacted by throwing her food around and hitting anyone who came near her. Mary got so upset that she reacted by yelling at her family. Often one of her daughters would storm off from the table in tears. It became obvious to Mary that this solution was not working for her and her family.

Mary's solution to the problem: *Mary thought about the three issues: her mother, her family, and her home. Mary decided to sit down with her daughters to come up with a strategy that would allow her family to share a meal together—a value that she considered very important.*

She sat down and talked with them. Mary explained to Lori and Beth why their grandmother needed to stay involved in family activities and why their actions caused Grandma to act out. Lori and Beth felt that Mary was being unreasonable by asking them to be quiet every night at dinner to avoid upsetting their grandmother. Mary explained a couple of things to them. First, it was important to her that their family share a meal together. Second, because of her dementia, her mother could not tolerate the over-stimulation caused by her granddaughters' music and bickering.

After discussing the situation with her daughters, Mary was able to reach a compromise with them. The whole family would share one meal a week together—usually Sunday breakfast. It was a less hectic time for Lori and Beth, and mornings were a quieter time for Mary's mother as well.

Once they understood this, Lori and Beth came up with a number of their own solutions to the problem. They were willing to assist Mrs. R. to set the table, put out the bread, and do other small mealtime tasks. They reduced the noise level in the house by choosing quiet, relaxing music and by turning off their cell phones. To make the occasion special, they decorated the table with flowers in an unbreakable vase. Sunday breakfast became a very important and meaningful time for the entire family. For dinner, Mary served Mrs. R. first and then later ate dinner with her daughters. This made the dinner much less stressful.

Eating together as a family may not be as important to you. In this situation, you might opt to feed your mother separately. It's up to you to choose a strategy and solutions that best fit in with *you* and *your* lifestyle.

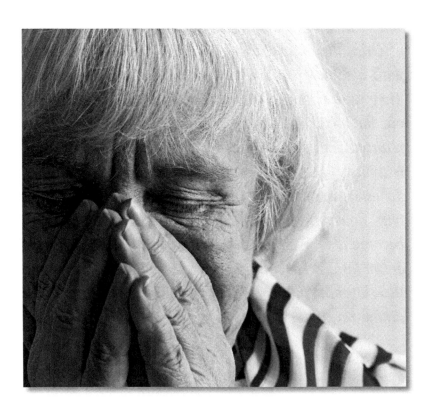

NOTES

_____

_____

_____

_____

_____

_____

_____

_____

_____

_____

_____

_____

_____

_____

_____

_____

_____

_____

_____

_____

_____

_____

_____

You were extremely helpful during a difficult time, and it helped my dad and my sisters to have your assessment added to the mix. My mom is safe, has a good routine, good care and the right nutrition. My dad has been able to calm down, semi-recoup, refocus on work. I am so grateful we found your organization and know that someday I will be sharing Memory Care Home Solutions as a resource with a friend or other family member. We will keep you posted on how things go, but for where we are right now, things are okay, and these days "okay" is the new "good."

— Stephanie, caregiver

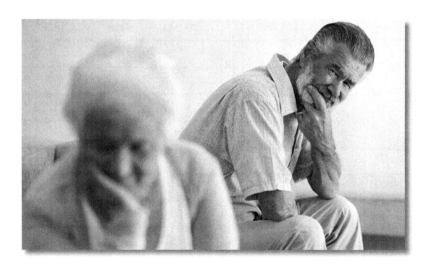

Who Did You Say You Were Again?
Understanding memory loss and dementia
and their impact on daily living

Is dementia the same as memory loss?

Age-related changes in cognition or thinking are common and are often experienced across the lifespan. Difficulty in coming up with a proper name, slowed reflexes or reaction time and, difficulty with multitasking, are all examples of age-related changes in cognition. These examples do not represent an underlying disease nor do they predict future deterioration or decline. In addition, these changes typically do not cause functional impairment.

Dementia on the other hand is often demonstrated by severe short-term memory loss where an individual will consistently forget conversations, repeat himself within minutes to hours, misplace items and may need assistance finding them, may forget events or the details of events, and may no longer be able to keep a calendar. These changes typically occur in the day-to-day life of the person and in personal, social or occupational settings. Instrumental activities of daily living such as driving, cooking and handling finances are frequently impaired in the early stages of the disease.

What is dementia?

Dementia is the name used to describe a set of recognizable symptoms that are associated with certain diseases or disorders of the brain. These symptoms get worse over time, and eventually interfere with a person's ability to perform his usual activities and care for himself. Symptoms of dementia include:

Memory loss, especially short-term memory loss. A person with dementia does not simply forget a word or misplace his keys every now and again. He will forget almost everything that has recently happened—a conversation he just had with you, the last meal he's eaten, a visit from a friend who went home fifteen minutes ago, and, eventually, even your name. While your husband can't remember the recent visit of a friend, he might be able to remember things that happened many years ago such as the names of all his childhood friends and where they lived. Long-term memory tends to remain intact for a longer period of time than short-term memory. People in the early stages are often very adept at covering up their memory loss, as the following story illustrates:

▪ Strategies & Solutions ▪

Bill's mom was always an immaculate woman and had a standing appointment every week with her hairdresser. He began to notice that her hair was messy and her gray roots were showing. When he confronted her about her appearance, she claimed that she had fired her hairdresser and had stopped going to the beauty salon entirely. Then he realized there was more to the story.

Bill's solution: A call to the receptionist revealed that his mom had missed five appointments in the past six months. It finally became clear to Bill that his mother was attempting to cover up her memory loss. He arranged a standing appointment for a time when he was able to bring her to the beauty salon and pick her up. Getting her hair done was a social occasion for her and she really enjoyed her time there. While she was having her hair done, he shopped and did chores for her.

Impairments in judgment: We all say and do inappropriate things at times, but people with dementia say and do more inappropriate things, more often. Your father may drive the wrong way on highways, urinate in a public flower bed, or say private or personal things to neighbors and acquaintances that he wouldn't normally say. Your mother might throw important papers into the garbage and give money away to someone who calls her on the phone.

▪ Strategies & Solutions ▪

Jan was the caregiver for her husband, Albert. As his dementia became worse, Albert started to curse at every little thing that bothered or annoyed him. At times, he even cursed at Jan and other family members. This was very upsetting to her as she was brought up to believe that cursing is a sin, something no nice person would do. But no matter how much she told Albert not to swear, it didn't seem to make any difference.

***Jan's Solutions:** Jan talked with her pastor. He told her that God would not condemn Albert for cursing because the disease robbed him of the capacity, or judgment, to recognize that what he did was not acceptable.*

First, Jan was able to ignore it because she knew Albert couldn't help himself and didn't really mean to hurt her. She came to recognize his cursing as a reaction to being upset. Second, because she could usually "see it coming" she could often distract him by putting on one of his favorite videos. He especially liked football and base-

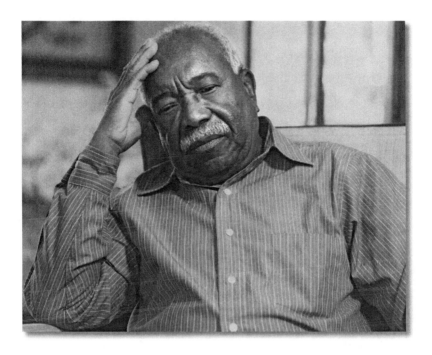

ball, and she taped the games and put them on whenever she needed to distract him. He no longer remembered the sequence of the game, or whether the game was live or not, but he enjoyed watching the action.

———————

Behavioral changes and fluctuating moods. Irritability, mood swings (depression alternating with extreme agitation), fear, and suspiciousness of everything and everybody are some of the changes that characterize dementia.

Some people with dementia are so terrified by the disease they unconsciously blame other people for what is happening to them. Your sister may accuse you, or the aide who helps with her care, of stealing her money when, in fact, she can't remember where she put it.

Dementia also peels away social behavior. Your mother may use sexual language that she wouldn't ordinarily use with you or your husband. The most mild-mannered man may scream and yell at you when he can't make himself understood.

▪ Strategies & Solutions ▪

Mrs. J. was in her sixties when she first became aware that something was wrong. A businesswoman, she was unable to complete business deals, do the math needed to create a simple bill, and drive to her business appointments. She alternated between sadness and depression at what she was no longer able to do. She also became agitated and angry when her husband tried to stop her from driving and to convince her to give up her business. She knew he was right, but giving up her independence was terrifying to her. She yelled at her husband who, as a result, became more and more withdrawn from her. As the dementia progressed, she became suspicious of her friends, who she claimed were siding with her husband, and she would also lash out at them.

Mr. J.'s solution: *The kinds of behavioral changes, which resulted from Mrs. J.'s fear and anxiety over what was happening to her, were very hard on Mr. J. and their friends. Mr. J. felt alienated from the woman he had always seen as his best friend. He decided to join an Alzheimer's support group where he learned that it was the disease process and his wife's reaction to it that were causing these kinds of changes in her behavior. Instead of feeling attacked and withdrawing from her, he learned to calmly respond to her anger. He was now able to explain the situation to their friends and help them remain supportive of his wife. The group also helped him mourn the woman she no longer was and accept the woman she had become—still his wife, but more limited.*

Failure to recognize familiar objects and faces. There will come a day when your mother doesn't just forget your name; she may well no longer recognize you, or your children. Your husband may look at a toothbrush, or a bar of soap, or his shoe and no longer remember what it is or what to do with it. A person with age-related memory loss may momentarily forget the word "toothbrush." But he will continue to know what it is and what to do with it. A person with dementia will gradually reach a point where he does not.

Problems with time, place, and person orientation. We all have moments when we don't quite know what day it is. People with dementia may no longer know what day it is even if you tell them. Your father may fail to remember his address or where he lives, and ultimately get to the point where he can't remember who he is.

▪ Strategies & Solutions ▪

Lila lived with her two sons and her father, George, who had Alzheimer's disease. On summer days, Lila liked to keep the front door open to allow her children to run in and out. But her father often left the house and wandered around the neighborhood. Frequently, he ended up at a house he had lived in many years ago, confused and upset because people he didn't know now lived there. (Returning to places familiar from the past often happens when people lose recent memory.) *Lila was embarrassed and anxious every time this happened until she learned of a program where the local police department would supply George with an ID bracelet that he couldn't remove. The bracelet gave his name, current address, and telephone number so that anyone finding him could telephone Lila to come and get him.* (If the police department in your community doesn't have such a program, you can buy a simple, inexpensive ID bracelet and have it engraved with the information.)

———————

Difficulties with understanding and expressing complex language. As dementia progresses, it becomes more and more difficult for the person who has it to understand what is said to them. As a result, they can't answer appropriately. Your sister may have problems following a simple conversation. She may look blankly when you ask her a question, or ignore the question and talk about something with which she is already familiar. Or she may repeat the same words and sentence fragments over and over again. (For further discussion about problems with language and communication, see Chapter 4.)

Problems with math calculations and simple reasoning. Dementia impairs a person's ability to think in the abstract, to do simple math, and to plan and organize everything from complex activities to daily tasks. Your husband can't balance his checkbook, your mother can't figure out what items to put on a shopping list, or your wife no longer knows that if she leaves perishable food out on a hot day it will spoil.

▪ Strategies & Solutions ▪

Joan's father, Roger, had been diagnosed with Alzheimer's disease two years ago. At that point he gave Joan power of attorney, but Roger was still able to take care of his monthly bills by noting on his calendar when the bills were due. One day, Joan tried to call her father and was shocked to realize that his phone had been disconnected. Joan found out that his line had been shut off because he had not paid his bill in two months. Although he was mailing the bills, he was not inserting checks.

__Joan's solution:__ At first she tried to go to his house once a month to assist him in paying his bills. But this reminder of his lost capacities upset Roger and he would accuse her of trying to take over his life and steal his money. Because she already had power of attorney, Joan was able to arrange to have the bills sent to her house where she paid them from their joint checking account.

Susceptibility to environmental over-stimulation. Most of us are able to perform tasks like washing dishes while the TV or radio is on, or while our children are talking to us, or we are talking on the phone. A person with dementia gradually loses the ability to do this.

They easily go into "stimulus overload" if there is too much going on in the environment around them. Think of a fuse box or a circuit breaker: If too many electrical appliances are running at one time, a fuse or circuit breaker will blow and everything on that line will shut down. If there is no fuse box or circuit breaker, the wire itself will start to burn. People with dementia have no self-regulating fuse box or circuit breaker. If too much is going on around them, they may "blow" and become extremely agitated and upset, and may even hit out or throw things at people. This is called a *catastrophic reaction*.

Reducing noise and over-stimulation in the environment, simplifying a complicated activity, or distracting them by gently removing them from the situation they find overwhelming and providing them with something they like such as a snack or favorite TV show, are a few ways to handle catastrophic reactions in people. Several of the case vignettes in the guidebook illustrate different solutions caregivers found to handle these outbursts. Once distracted, they will most likely forget about being upset quite quickly.

Is dementia the same as Alzheimer's disease?

Dementia is an umbrella term used to describe a set of mental functioning deficits that get worse over time.

There are many forms of dementia and they can be caused by different conditions. Alzheimer's disease is the most common form. Other causes of dementia include Parkinson's disease, multi-infarct or vascular (stroke), head trauma, AIDS-related dementia, frontal-temporal, Lewy body (the second most common form of dementia), and late-stage alcoholism or Wernike-Korsakoff.

Is dementia ever reversible?

Some dementias such as those produced by over-medication, malnourishment, tumors, thyroid issue, vitamin deficiencies, depression, and infections are reversible with treatment. Dementias caused by Alzheimer's disease, vascular problems, late-stage alcoholism, and other disease processes are chronic and not reversible with treatment. In fact, they usually get worse over time. It is important for the person with suspected dementia to have a thorough physical evaluation that includes a full range of diagnostic tests, such as brain and blood work, to rule out any of the reversible conditions. Over-medication is a particular issue for older people and will often cause dementia-like symptoms. If you suspect your mother may have dementia and want to take her to the doctor, put all her medications into a paper bag and bring it along to the doctor's office so these medications, their side-effects, and their interactions can be evaluated. The doctor will begin to rule out any other issues before giving a dementia diagnosis. Remember that the sooner you have an accurate diagnosis, the sooner proper treatment can begin.

Putting it into practice

Think about the person with dementia you are caring for.

- What kinds of problems do they experience as a result of the dementia?

- What is the impact of these problems on you and your family?

- Can you think of a simple solution to one problem you listed that could be helped by gently removing them from the situation causing the trouble or outburst and focusing their attention on something they enjoy (distraction)?

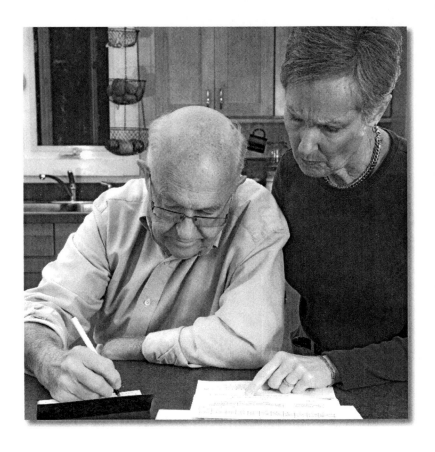

NOTES

Dear Steve:

I must tell you that I think Bill is trying very hard and really has only given me static (and only for about five minutes) once since your visit. Something about me moving his keys.

I asked him to check around as I didn't have them. After about five minutes it dawned on me that they could be in the pair of trousers he last wore. Sure enough, and he seemed grateful and is placing his keys on the table. This may sound trivial to you, but it's a major milestone for us.

Per your letter, I will not load him down with plans or schedules until closer to the dates involved. This will really simplify things for us.

We did get a cordless phone from last Thursday and so far so good. I've called him from church on Saturday and he was able to answer and didn't seem intimidated. It has two receivers and a paging system.

I so appreciate your visit and feel relieved that you're out there for us.

— Loretta

I'd Rather Do It Myself
Planning and adapting daily activities

Supporting and maintaining remaining capacities

Although people with dementia may act in childlike ways at times, it is important to remember that they are still adults. As adults we all have the same basic needs for independence, times of activity and rest, love and affection, feelings of self-worth, respect, and esteem.

Maintaining independence

Unlike children who are moving from dependence to independence, people with Alzheimer's disease are moving from independence to dependence as the disease process strips them of their abilities to meet their basic needs. Much depends on *you*, the caregiver, to help the person you are caring for maintain her ability to meet her needs in a way that reflects the person she has been and, in many ways, still is. One way to do this is to help her retain her functional abilities for as long as possible.

What is "functional ability?"

Functioning means that a person has both the **ability** and **willingness** to perform tasks and activities. Your mother may want to make fried chicken for the family, but does she remember how to do it? In other words, does she still have the ability to complete the many steps involved in preparing fried chicken? Your father may still have the ability to mow the lawn in that he *remembers* how to do it, but does he *want* to mow the lawn? In other words, does he have the willingness to do it? Dementia limits people's **ability** to do things, especially complicated things. It may seem like they don't want to do something when, in fact, they are no longer able to do it. (See Chapter 2 for a further discussion of what dementia is and how it affects people.)

Ability vs. willingness

While your mother may have the ability to perform small tasks like dipping the chicken pieces into the crumbs, does she have the willingness or motivation to do it? People with dementia have many feelings about having the condition. They may become depressed and feel as though the disease has already taken away so much from them—why even bother to keep trying? Other people may become anxious and frustrated with themselves at not being able to do it, or do it as well as they once did, and give up before they start. By using some of the strategies and solutions suggested in this chapter and in the rest of the guidebook, you may be able to lessen some of these feelings and/or motivate them to keep trying. But some people may need professional help. If you believe that the person you are caring for is very depressed or anxious, set up an appointment with a doctor, or a good mental health practitioner. Depression and anxiety are treatable conditions and even people with dementia can be helped to feel better.

If you don't use it, you lose it

When a person with dementia continues to stay involved in daily life, to function as best they can in their self-care activities, to do a piece of a task even if they can't do the whole thing, his brain stays active and he loses functioning ability at a slower rate than people who don't stay physically and mentally active. As you read on in this chapter, you will learn how to simplify daily activities to help the person for whom you are caring stay involved and active for as long as possible.

Maintaining dignity and self-worth

In our lives, adults are expected to be able to care for themselves and most adults want to do this. Although dementia progressively limits your brother's functional ability, there are many ways in which he can continue to participate in his daily routines, as this chapter will show you. Your brother's continued participation in daily life activities allows him to maintain dignity and self-worth.

Maintaining involvement in social and family life

With few exceptions, most people need to feel loved and cared about, and they need to love back. Under the right conditions, people with dementia can still be a part of social and family life. Your mother, who may no longer be able to read a daily newspaper, may be able to teach your little daughter the nursery rhymes that she still remembers from long ago. Your poker-playing father may not be the whiz he once was, but he may still be able to enjoy playing a simple game of War or Match the Cards with you if nobody really cares much about following the rules. *Just remember that people with dementia can't adapt to the needs of others; you and your family must understand and adapt to theirs.*

Change is the name of the game

Over time, dementia wears away more and more of people's functional abilities. Your mother may be able to set the table with very little assistance now. Six months from now, she may forget which utensils to

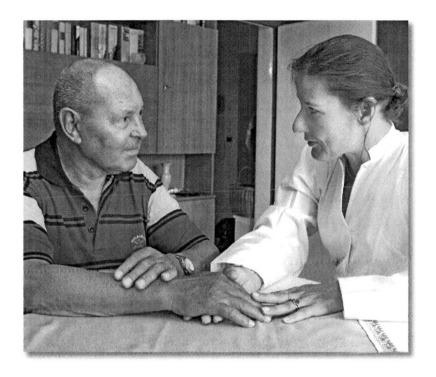

set out without being reminded. Your husband may know how to shave himself today. Three months or six months from now, he may need you to remind him how to work the nozzle of the shaving cream can. Be aware of the increasing limitations of the person you are caring for, and be prepared to offer more assistance as necessary.

Isn't it easier to just do it myself?
There's no doubt that some of the suggestions in this chapter for simplifying activities will take time and

effort on your part. You may feel that it's easier and less stressful to just do it yourself. For example, if you are rushing out of the house, you may not have the time to help your husband put on his clothes; you may elect to do it for him. But at another time, when you aren't so rushed, you may have the time to guide him to dress himself, set the table, shave himself, or participate in other activities. Allowing the person with dementia to take an active role in tasks provides him with feelings of purpose and self-worth.

Be creative in your approach

There are many ways to help people with dementia continue to stay involved in daily activities and do things for themselves, and not every suggestion in this chapter will be right for everyone. The key is to be creative and to not give up. If one way doesn't work, try something else.

■ Strategies & Solutions ■

Carl, a 68-year-old man with arthritis and early-stage dementia caused by a stroke, refused to take showers. His wife, Beth, tried everything, but nothing worked.

Beth's solution: After weeks of frustration she happened to mention this problem to their physician during a routine office visit of her own. The physician wrote an actual prescription for showers and gave it to Carl during his next office visit. Each time Carl was resistant to the idea of showering, Beth showed him the doctor's order stating that he take a hot shower each day to relieve his arthritis. Lo and behold, his doctor could make him do what his wife could not!

This chapter will teach you many strategies and solutions to help you keep the person you are caring for involved in more activities, more of the time. The goal is to increase the overall amount of time and ways the person you are caring for can be involved in activities of daily life. But there will always be situations when you will be feeling too rushed, too harried, or too frustrated to handle the helping role with calm and patience, and you will choose to do it yourself. Don't feel guilty. There's always the next time.

Planning daily activities

The key to helping a person with dementia remain as functional as possible is to plan in advance. Here are some tips:

1. Establish a structured daily routine. A regular daily schedule for such things as getting up, eating, bathing, grooming, dressing, napping, and going to bed helps to minimize confusion and behavior problems. Routines establish familiar patterns. These patterns can make certain tasks less fearful, lower anxiety, and provide needed structure for both the person with memory loss and the caregiver.

▪ Strategies & Solutions ▪

Lois was a caregiver to her mother, Eleanor. From time to time, Lois would take her mother out shopping. During or after these outings, Eleanor would become agitated, either stomping her feet and shaking her fists, or pacing around the house. Lois knew it was important for her mother to get out, but realized that her mother became anxious about changes in her familiar routine. The agitation was her mother's way of expressing her anxiety.

Lois' solution: *She took her mother out shopping daily. This made it part of her mother's daily routine and reduced her agitation. These outings then became a familiar part of her routine, and Eleanor looked forward to them.*

2. Incorporate old habits and preferences. Consider the preferences of the person for whom you are providing care, not *your own* preferences when you are establishing a routine. If your mother always took a shower before going to bed, continuing with that pattern will also minimize confusion and help her feel more like her old self. Incorporating relaxing activities that your mother always enjoyed into her routine may also help reduce agitation and other disruptive behaviors. Engaging your mother in meaningful activities can reduce unwanted behavior and will give her a sense of purpose.

▪ Strategies & Solutions ▪

Bill, a 74-year-old man with dementia who was cared for by his son, Robert, paced back and forth frequently throughout the day. When Robert would ask what he was doing, Bill would answer, "You know what I'm looking for." Of course Bob didn't know what his father was looking for; he just knew he was agitated.

Bob's solution: *Memory Care Home Solutions' social worker, Steve, recommended that Bob purchase a recliner for his father and give him a music player with headphones to listen to his favorite hymns. The comfortable* *chair and the music created something familiar for his father. These solutions helped him relax and he began to pace less often.*

---

3. Post the schedule. Write each day's schedule of activities on a large piece of paper or whiteboard with dry erase markers. This provides a reference for other family members and paid caregivers.

4. Be flexible and willing to compromise. Structure is important, but too much insistence upon routine can lead to agitation and other undesirable behaviors. People with dementia have moods, just as we all do. Your husband may feel a little lethargic one day, or have a cold coming on and be unable to tell you about it. He may not feel like doing his exercises, or be unwilling to take a bath in the morning. If you insist, he may become agitated or upset. Since he can't explain his feelings, you have to learn to "read" him. Try suggesting a bath later in the day or see if he feels a little more energetic then. If he still is unwilling, don't try to force him, or press him too hard. Try again the next day.

Modifying activities

Most activities that people enjoy doing consist of multiple steps. Think about frying chicken. If you've fried chicken all your life, it may seem simple to you. But there are actually many steps involved in doing it.

- Purchasing the chicken (shopping)

- Bringing it home (knowing how to travel and remembering where you live)

- Assembling the ingredients (remembering what you need to make fried chicken and being able to locate these ingredients in the cupboard)

- Remembering the order of steps that go into preparing the chicken (washing the chicken, patting it dry, dipping it in milk or egg, dipping it in crumbs)

- Knowing how to work the stove, heat the oil, time the cooking, etc.

Your mother may not be able to plan and organize this complicated series of steps, but she may be able to do one or two of the steps with some help.

▪ Strategies & Solutions ▪

Sarah, who has moderate-stage dementia, used to love gardening but could no longer care for the large flower garden in her back yard. Instead, she'd sit in her chair, staring out the window at the garden and rocking back and forth. Jane, her daughter, knew how much her mother missed her old activity.

Jane's solutions: *Here are some solutions that helped Jane modify gardening activities for her mother:*

1. *Jane decided what gardening activities her mother could still do with some help. She believed that Sarah could still dig up the ground to prepare it for planting and that she could probably dig a hole with some help and place a plant in the hole.*

2. *Jane planned ahead and had everything her mother needed ready to go.*

3. *She handed Sarah a small garden fork and showed her where the ground needed loosening.*

4. *Sarah was able to loosen the soil, but she had forgotten how to dig a hole for the plant. Jane demonstrated how*

to dig the hole. Her mother was then able to dig several holes.

5. *Jane handed her one plant and Sarah popped it right into the hole.*

6. *After Sarah had done this several times, she began to rock back and forth in an agitated way. Jane realized she was tired and had reached her limit. So they stopped. But Sarah was happy for the rest of the day.*

7. *The next day Sarah was ready to garden once more. Jane had to coach her again because Sarah had forgotten the steps.*

Simplify, simplify

Think of the steps involved in completing an activity as the "recipe" for that task. Then look for ways to make each step as simple as possible. Continually ask yourself, "How can I make this easier?"

Here are some more examples:

- Select finger foods at meal times to eliminate the use of a fork and knife.

- Use Velcro fasteners, which are easier to close than buttons or snaps.

- Choose self-stick pictures for creating collages rather than ones that need glue.

Limit or eliminate choices

Even though someone with dementia can have preferences, having too many choices at one time is confusing. Simplify choices by selecting something and then asking him if he'd like to do it. For example, don't ask your husband if he wants to wear the white shirt or the brown shirt. Give him the white shirt and say, "Would you like to wear this shirt?" If he says no, then take out the tan shirt, give it him, and ask him if he'd like to wear the tan shirt.

Communicate what you're doing while you're doing it

While complex language skills may be lost, people with dementia may still be able to understand and enjoy simple "talk" and find it comforting and soothing. Take your cue from the person; if your "talk" seems to agitate her, use simpler language—one or two words—and just don't expect too much back in the way of conversation. (See Chapter 4 for ways to improve your ability to communicate with people who have dementia.)

▪ Strategies & Solutions ▪

Jill R. was the caregiver to her husband, Lenny. Lenny could still dress himself with Jill's assistance, but the whole process got him very agitated. Lenny would often yell at Jill, and several times hit her when she handed him his clothes to put on.

Jill's solution: *Jill found that talking to Lenny in a gentle, conversational tone about what she was doing while she was doing it reduced his agitation. For example, she would smile and say, "Here's your shirt, Honey, just out of the wash." He put it on. Then she handed him his pants, and continued the conversation but kept it simple, saying: "Here are the black pants you like." Lenny responded to her calm, conversational manner by staying calm himself and getting dressed.*

Putting it into practice

Think of an activity that the person you are caring for has always enjoyed doing but that has now become a little too complicated. Briefly review the steps necessary to complete the activity. Then:

- Select one or two steps or a portion of the activity that you think the person can still do.

- Decide what you will need to have prepared in advance for the person to be able to complete the one or two steps you selected. *Remember, keep it simple and at the functional level of the person who will do the activity.*

- Try it out and see what happens. Did you make the activity simple enough? Too simple? What, if anything, will you do differently next time?

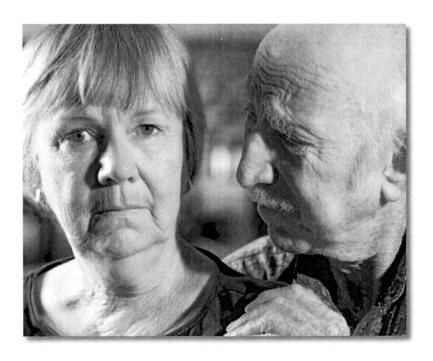

I'd Rather Do It Myself

NOTES

71

My seven sisters and brothers never thought that our mother would need our care. Our mom's body is still here but much of who she was is gone. As Mom's condition worsened my father, my siblings and myself were all searching for answers as to how best to help her and to cope with the sadness of losing our mom before our eyes. Truthfully, we were all going in opposite directions.

Steve compassionately instructed us on the stages of Mom's disease and the changing methods of care that we will have to implement in the future.

Sincerely,
— Michelle

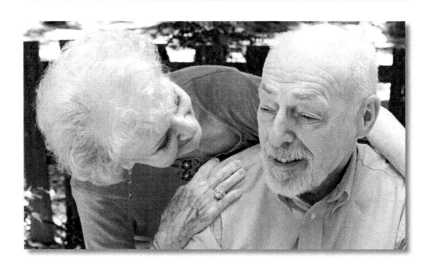

Talking the Talk
Communicating with people who have memory loss and impaired language

People in the moderate stages of dementia experience many problems with using and understanding language. Your wife may have a hard time remembering the names of things, may easily lose the thread of a conversation, may be unable to remember simple instructions, and may ask the same question repeatedly because she doesn't remember what she's just said, or the answer you've given.

Adapting to language limitations

When communicating with a person who has dementia, you must adapt to his limitations. Language problems differ from person to person, from day to day, and from moment to moment. People with dementia have good days and bad days. On good days, your father may be able to understand a little better and respond more fully. On bad days—days that he is feeling frustrated, upset, anxious, or tired—his ability to understand and respond may be less. Don't assume that just because your father can tell you what he wants for dinner one day, that he will be able to tell you the next. Make it a point to tune into his mood and language ability each time you talk to him, and adjust your conversational style and expectations accordingly.

The importance of non-verbal communication

All communication consists of two parts:

- **verbal:** the spoken word
- **non-verbal:** gestures, facial expressions, body language, touch, and tone of voice

People with dementia have a harder time understanding and using verbal language, so it is important to tune into and use non-verbal communication.

Tips for tuning into and using non-verbal language

- **Become aware of your non-verbal communication:** touch, tone of voice, facial expressions, and gestures, and use it to reinforce your words.

- **Learn to "read" the non-verbal messages your mother is sending you.** Her facial expressions and/or tone of voice will let you know if she is upset or anxious, or doesn't understand what you are saying.

- **Be aware of what you are feeling when you are speaking.** If you are feeling angry, even if it isn't directed at her, it might make her feel anxious or threatened. Try to calm down before speaking, and approach her in a gentle, reassuring manner.

- **Establish and maintain good eye contact.** This is calming and reassuring and will help you to get your message across more easily.

- **Use gestures to reinforce and clarify your words.** For example, if you want her to put her shoes on, say it, and mime the act of putting on a shoe if she still doesn't understand.

■ Strategies & Solutions ■

Debbie B. is the caregiver to her father, Frank, who has Alzheimer's disease. She wants to get her father ready to go to church, but she is having a bad day. Her teenage son has been acting up, she had an argument with her sister who thinks that Debbie is "babying" Frank too much, and Debbie has had it! Debbie approaches her father with her hands on her hips and a scowl on her face and says, "Come on, Dad. It's time to get ready to go to church." Frank immediately feels as if he is in trouble and is confused as to what made Debbie angry. As a result, Frank gets angry and agitated and pushes her away.

Debbie's solutions: *Debbie realized she had to reduce her own stress and anger before she approached her father. First, she tried counting to ten and taking deep breaths. Second, she visualized a duck looking calm and beautiful as it swims along the surface of the water (even though it may be kicking and paddling furiously underneath). The next Sunday she was able to approach her father calmly, with a smile on her face. She rubbed his hand and said gently, "Dad, let's get ready to go to church." This tone and expression told Frank that Debbie was not angry at him, that she is a cheerful and reassuring person, and that he can trust her.*

Reduce environmental distractions

Be aware of environmental distractions. These may include:

- A loud radio or TV
- Too dim or too bright lighting
- Multiple people speaking at once
- Large groups

These environmental distractions are confusing, create communication barriers, and cause anxiety for people with dementia.

Remember the 4 S's—simple, short, slow, and specific

When speaking to a person with dementia, remember to keep it **simple**, keep it **short**, keep it **slow**, and be **specific**. Here's how to do it:

Simple: Break sentences and instructions into their simplest components. State each idea or step in a task and check for understanding before going on to the next one. For example, when it is time for your wife to go out:

1. Put her coat in her hand. Gently and calmly say, "Here's your coat. Put it on now."

2. Wait until she's put on her coat before you give her the hat.

3. Walk over to the door with her, smile, and say, "Let's go out now."

4. Always check her facial expressions and body language to see whether she has understood. Take your cue from her.

5. Avoid using the phrase, "Don't you remember?" If she could remember, she would. Simply repeat the instruction again in a calm, reassuring voice.

Short: Use short sentences that don't contain a lot of complicated information. For example, if it is dinner time, say "It's time to eat," rather than "It's time to eat, and we are having chicken, and you know how much you love chicken, especially the way I fry it." This is too much information and can cause your mother to become frustrated, confused, or agitated.

Slow: Speak slowly. It takes time for people with dementia to process what you've said. Your father is more likely to get the message if you speak slowly, clearly, and calmly. And allow sufficient time for him to respond before you make the next statement.

Specific: Tell your wife specifically what you want her to do, in positive rather than negative terms. Here are some examples:

1. "Put on your slip" is better than "Don't put your slip on over your dress like you did last time."

2. "Here is your sweater" is better than "Don't you want to wear your sweater?" This could be interpreted by someone with dementia to mean that you don't want her to wear her sweater.

3. Avoid asking general questions such as "What do you want for lunch?" Be specific. Here is an example:

- "We are having pizza."
- If your sister doesn't want pizza, make another suggestion: "We can have scrambled eggs."
- If you must ask a question, make it specific: "Do you want scrambled eggs?" is better than "What would you rather have, pizza or scrambled eggs?"

4. Tell her what she can do, not what she cannot do. For example, if she is going into a room that is off limits, then gently redirect her to an area that is safe and find an activity she can do.

Use distraction and reassurance

If your husband is upset about something, don't try to explain or argue—this is using a logic that he can no longer understand. Instead, reassure him by saying, "It's okay. Everything will be fine." Then, distract him with something he likes—a favorite snack or a musical selection. Most likely, he will forget what he was upset about just a few minutes before.

Don't keep answering the same question

If your sister goes on asking the same question again and again ("Is Johnny coming today?") and you've already answered it several times already, stop answering it. She may simply be worried or upset. Instead, give her a hug or say in a reassuring voice, "It's okay, I'll tell you as soon as Johnny gets here." Then distract her with something that she likes.

And finally: These are suggestions only. Take your cues from the person you are caring for. Your wife will let you know which strategies work for her and which ones don't. Remember, "change" is the name of the game. What works one day may not work the next. Most important: be flexible and don't give up.

▪ Strategies & Solutions ▪

Frank's wife, Margaret, had Alzheimer's disease. He helped her dress herself by approaching her calmly, maintaining good eye contact, and using short, simple sentences to help her follow each step. As the disease progressively worsened, she started to resist him and would not dress herself. Frank got increasingly frustrated. One day, he decided to just let her wear her pajamas all day rather than go through another bout of frustration.

One morning as Frank was getting dressed, Margaret started to dress herself also. Amazed, he realized that she could copy his actions although she could no longer follow the simple verbal commands he had been using. From then on, he did not tell her to get dressed. He simply laid out her clothes and as he removed his pajamas and dressed himself, she followed his actions.

Putting it into practice

Think about a recent conversation or interaction with the person you are providing care for that didn't turn out well or caused problems.

- Were there any distractions going on while you were trying to talk to him? For example: Was the TV on? Were there other conversations going on in the room?

- What kind of language problems was he having in trying to talk to you? For example: Did he forget words? Did he use the wrong word to describe something? Did he repeat the same question again and again? Did he not pay attention to what you were trying to tell him?

- How did you feel about this conversation? For example: Did you feel angry, frustrated or annoyed?

- During a future conversation with this person, try to remember the 4 S's and keep it simple, short, slow, and specific. Ask yourself afterwards if the conversation went better, or if anything was improved.

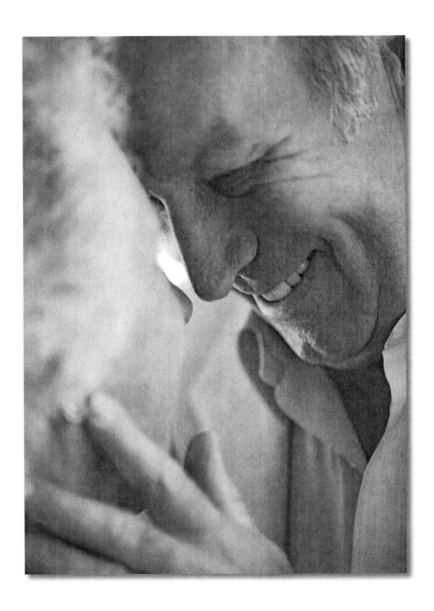

NOTES

After you left I took a more critical look at my house. I couldn't believe that I found samples of medication, two starter pistols and several pocket knives in the drawer of his nightstand. It never occurred to me to look in there as our night stands were more or less our own. Also in the back of the closet were a shotgun and a 22 rifle that I'd completely forgotten about. I had my son come and take them away. I am an excellent shot but I don't think it's safe for Glenn to have guns in the house.

I bought locks for cabinets and caps for doorknobs. I couldn't find any yellow tape in the store so I'll just use paint on a warmer day for the step in the garage.

Thanks for sending me your report. I can't tell you what a tremendous help you've been to us.

Thanks again,
— Doris

5

Home Sweet Home — with Dementia:
Modifying the home environment
to optimize functioning[1]

One of the most important things you can do when caring for someone with Alzheimer's disease at home is to
create an environment that compensates for the deficits
the disease produces. The following suggestions run
the gamut from the simple to the more complicated,
and range in cost from inexpensive to expensive. It is
up to you to decide which modifications meet your
needs and your budget.

Suggestions for home modifications
Lighting
People with Alzheimer's disease can have trouble making sense of what they are seeing. Daylight is the most
comfortable kind of light for them. Glare and shadows
are distracting and confusing. To create indoor light-

---

1 The content for this chapter has been adapted from Joanne Koenig
Coste, *Learning to Speak Alzheimer's*. Houghton Mifflin, 2003.

ing that better enhances functioning, consider making some of the following modifications:

- Replace regular bulbs with bulbs that mimic daylight such as "Vita Lights" or "Day Glow."

- Reduce the number of lamps in a room. Too many lamps create too many shadows, which people with dementia can find threatening.

- Light the path to the bathroom. Run a path of sticky-backed reflector tape from the bedroom to the bathroom, illuminating it with several nightlights. You may be able to reduce or eliminate nighttime accidents.

- Dimmer switches can be installed and turned up as the sun begins to set. This may help a person with Sundowners Syndrome. This syndrome, characterized by agitation, becomes evident from 3:00 p.m. to 8:00 p.m.

- Try to replace floor lamps with wall or ceiling lights to reduce clutter and make moving around the room easier and safer.

Color schemes

Alzheimer's disease affects people's reactions to color. People with the disease have difficulty selecting objects that are similarly colored, or can feel afraid and confused by too many colors and patterns. When used together, lighter shades, such as beige on white, do not provide enough contrast. They blend into each other and can cause people to feel disoriented. You can use color to enhance functioning in the following ways:

- Use flat rather than high-gloss paint on walls to reduce glare and shadows.

- Use specific, bright colors for different areas and spaces. For example, a sitting or TV area can be painted one bright color. The food preparation area can be painted another bright color. This can help orient people and enable them to move from one room to another without getting lost.

- Use wall colors that contrast with functional objects in a room. For example: if furniture is dark wood, paint the walls a light color. The use of bright colors, such as in colorful cushions on dining room chairs and on place mats, can help draw attention to an object and jog one's memory as to where to sit for meals.

- Put a piece of same-colored tape on objects that are used for one activity, such as hobby materials or grooming implements. This can cue an individual with dementia to help him remember that these materials are used together.

- Place a black mat in front of the door to keep a person from wandering into areas that may contain harmful objects, such as the front yard, laundry room, or pantry. The color black on a floor is perceived as a dark hole. When people with dementia encounter a black mat, they will often turn around and go the other way.

- Avoid contrasting stripes, polka dots, and checks because they increase visual confusion.

▪ Strategies & Solutions ▪

As Gary's father's dementia became more severe, he lost the ability to distinguish between the toilet and the floor because both were the same color. As a result, he constantly urinated on the floor instead of the toilet.

Gary's solution: *He placed a blue wrap-around rug in front of the toilet and fastened it to the floor with Velcro* *tape. The difference in color helped his father to distinguish between the floor and toilet.*

———————

Flooring
Many people with dementia walk with a shuffling gait because the disease affects balance. To help prevent falls, you can do the following:

- Try to keep linoleum or tile surfaces clean and dull rather than shiny. Shine produces glare, which can be confusing and distracting.

- Eliminate scatter or area rugs, which can cause accidents and falls.

- Repair or level uneven flooring.

- Try to use light-colored flooring material, if possible, since it tends to make a space seem larger and less confining.

Interior pathways
Colorful wallpaper borders or reflective tape placed at waist height can establish clear pathways between frequently used areas such as bedroom-to-bathroom

and bedroom-to-kitchen. Continue the tape or border across unsafe doorways (which should be kept closed). When your husband thinks a door is part of a wall, he will probably not attempt to open it.

Furniture and wall decorations

- Eliminate furniture that is wobbly or from which it is difficult to get in and out. Replace with sturdy chairs that: 1) are not too low to the ground, 2) have arms to push up from, and 3) are not backward-tilting.

- Porch gliders that do not lift off the floor can be soothing and relaxing. Rocking chairs, on the other hand, tend to be unsafe.

- Built-in shelves are safer than free-standing units.

- Mirrors should be removed as the disease progresses because they can cause confusion and upset people who no longer recognize their own image. Replace with a different wall decoration.

- Replace reflective glass over pictures and photographs with no-glare glass.

- Wall décor should be soothing and comforting. Some examples are: simple pictures of favorite scenes, children's artwork, and textured fabric hangings such as a piece of soft carpet that can be stroked or touched.

- Eliminate reminders of hobbies that people can no longer enjoy. Encourage more simple hobbies and keep their tools or components in plain view and in separate compartments, such as a silverware tray, to provide easy access and avoid confusion.

- Install a sturdy fish tank and fill it with some colorful fish. (You'll have to establish and control the feeding schedule so the fish don't get fed too often, but a comfortable chair placed in front of the tank will provide many calm and happy hours for your father.)

Using pictures instead of words

As memory and language become less usable, use pictures and images of items to replace words. Some suggestions:

- Tape a picture of dishes on the door of the appropriate cabinet.

- Place a picture of panties or a bra on the underwear drawer.

- Tape a picture of a toilet on the bathroom door, or on the wall next to the door if you plan to leave it open.

▪ Strategies & Solutions ▪

1. Kathleen's mother had moderate stage of Alzheimer's disease and Kathleen realized that her mother was throwing dirty toilet paper in the hamper instead of the toilet.

Kathleen's solutions: *First, she removed the hamper from the bathroom. Next, she taped a large picture above the toilet that showed a hand dropping toilet paper in the toilet.*

2. Gordon's father, who had dementia because of a stroke, began using the hallway trash can as a toilet.

Gordon's solutions: *First, he removed all trash cans that were located near the bathroom. Then, he taped a large picture of a toilet on the bathroom door.*

Both of these solutions involved two steps: the first was to remove the item that was inappropriately used for the real thing (the toilet); the second was to use a picture of the real thing as a memory cue.

Safety devices

Many devices exist to increase safety of the environment of a person with Alzheimer's disease. You can try some of the following safety devices. Sometimes you might have to experiment with different ones.

- Install child safety gates at the top and the bottom of stairs.

- Install a hook-and-eye type fastener near the top or the bottom of doors that you don't want opened. People with Alzheimer's disease most likely won't look in improbable places for these items.

■ Strategies & Solutions ■

Paul had mid-stage Alzheimer's disease. He lived with his daughter, Mary, and her son, Jimmy. Mary was his full-time caregiver. Paul was starting to wander outside of the home. There had been a few times when Mary had been upstairs and had not heard Paul leave through the front door.

Mary's solutions: *Mary first installed a hook-and-eye fastener near the top of the door, but her son, Jimmy, couldn't reach it to get out. Jimmy liked to run outside to greet his friends when they came over to play. He became upset when he couldn't get the door open. The Memory Care Home Solutions social worker, Steve, recommended that Mary install door alarms that were controlled by a remote, which Jimmy could operate. He turned it off when he ran out to meet his friends, and turned it on when they came in. Mary felt comfortable knowing that if her father wandered out the front door, she was able to hear the alarm.*

————————

- Install childproof locks on closet doors and drawers that contain potentially harmful items such as medical or cleaning supplies. Install childproof locks on any other closets that you don't want explored.

- Consult your local gas company on ways to make your gas oven or stove tamper-proof.

- Install safety bars in tubs and showers for people with balance problems.

▪ Strategies & Solutions ▪

As the caregiver for his wife, Betty, John needed to continually remind her to turn off the water after she washed her hands. The sink overflowed many times because Betty did not turn off the water and she would fall on the slick floor. This became a huge safety issue. John put up signs showing a hand turning the water off, but Betty did not understand these signs.

***John's solution:** John installed automatic shut-off faucets. The installation of the new faucets made it possible for Betty to continue using the sink and he stopped worrying that it was going to overflow.*

Putting it into practice
Think about your own home.
- What kind of obstacles or limitations does your home create for the person for whom you provide care for?

- List some simple modifications you could undertake that would make your home safer, more secure, and less stressful for that person.

- Choose the two or three that would be the easiest and most useful to undertake.

- Make a commitment to yourself to make these modifications in your home.

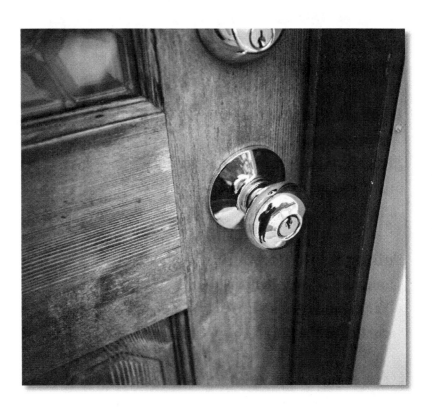

NOTES

Recently my husband became agitated with me because I would not let him take the trash out, something he wants to do anytime he sees a piece of trash in the can. During his agitated state, he began choking me. He let me go pretty quickly, but I was scared. After talking with my social worker, I learned a few new strategies. I'm now keeping the trash cans hidden until after dinner, then he can take them out. I'm also letting him take out the trash earlier in the day too. This makes him feel good, but now it's not all day long.

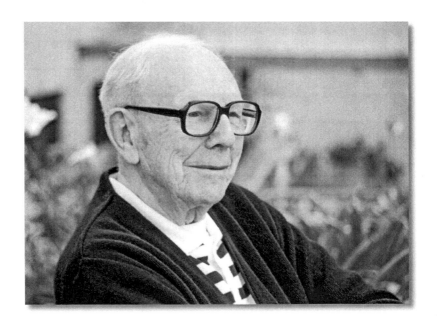

Anywhere I Wander
Managing disruptive behaviors in the home

Knowing which behaviors can and can't be managed

There are two broad categories of behavior problems associated with dementia. The first category includes problems that can't be cured or reduced and tend to get worse as the disease progresses. Examples are:

- progressive loss of ability to use language to communicate complex ideas
- progressive loss of ability to recognize familiar objects
- meaningless repetition of actions or sounds

The second category includes certain problems that not everyone with dementia will exhibit, but that many do. They can be controlled or lessened by simple activities and environmental modifications. Three of these behavioral problems will be discussed in this chapter, along with some solutions for controlling or lessening them. If other family members either live with you or are involved in providing care, it is important to share this information with them so that they will understand these behaviors and be able to deal with them also.

Sundowners Syndrome

Sundowners Syndrome is defined as confusion, agitation, or restlessness that occurs in the late afternoon or early evening. It can be aggravated by stressful situations or environments. These may include too many people, loud radios, TVs and noisy computer or video games, and other environmental distractions. (See Chapter 1 for further discussion about environmental over-stimulation.)

▪ Strategies & Solutions ▪

Mr. B: A description of Sundowners Syndrome

Mrs. B. cares for her husband who has Alzheimer's disease. While she had always enjoyed watching TV as she cooked, this activity has now become the most dreaded part of her day. Although Mr. B. has always had a rather calm disposition, since he developed Alzheimer's, he has become increasingly agitated during the late afternoon and early evening, just when Mrs. B. is preparing dinner. He paces back and forth through the apartment and gets easily upset. He can no longer do the activities that Mrs. B. sets up for him. The entire situation makes Mrs. B. so angry and frustrated that she often ends up in tears.

———————

Managing Sundowners Syndrome

Here are some simple environmental modifications and changes in the couple's activity patterns and schedules that might help Mrs. B. control or lessen her husband's Sundowners Syndrome.

Mrs. B. might consider:

- preparing dinner earlier in the day when her husband doesn't need as much of her attention, or can tolerate a little more distraction.

- creating a calm environment by taping sporting events and watching them earlier in the day or playing classical or easy-listening music (more soothing to a person with Sundowners Syndrome) during late afternoons.

- scheduling more physical activities such as walks and exercise earlier in the day in order to tire her husband out and expend his energy.

Other things that you might try if the person you are caring for has Sundowners Syndrome:

- schedule necessary activities such as bathing and medical appointments for earlier in the day
- surround the person you are caring for with familiar and beloved objects
- encourage afternoon naps to reduce fatigue and agitation

Wandering

Wandering is a common behavioral problem experienced by many people with dementia. You probably cannot eliminate it completely, but you can manage it by reducing the potential dangers involved and creating an environment in which it is safe to wander.

People with dementia wander for different reasons. Family caregivers try to figure out what their loved one needs because he no longer knows how to ask for it. Ask yourself: Does the person I'm caring for want something? Does he need to go the bathtoom? Is he hungry? Has he lost or misplaced something? He may also wander because he is simply bored, upset, or over-stimulated.

▪ Strategies & Solutions ▪

Clara, who has moderate-stage dementia, was always an active woman. Two years ago, she went to live with her son, Will, and his wife, who both worked full time. Being alone all day caused Clara to become extremely bored and restless. When Will checked on her during his lunch break, he always found her pacing through the house. When he asked her what she was doing, she would reply, "I don't know."

Will's solution: *Will enrolled his mother in an adult day center. The structured activities at the adult day care reduced her agitation. In the evenings, when both he and his wife were home, Clara was calm.*

Managing or reducing wandering behaviors
If an adult day-care center is not a choice for you, here are some things you might do to manage or reduce wandering behaviors in the home:
- remind the person to go to the bathroom every couple of hours
- reduce noise, distractions, and lights to minimize stress
- provide a distracting activity—a walk, favorite music, a stuffed animal for cuddling

- leave lights on at night
- mark the route from bedroom to bathroom with a strip of contrasting-color tape
- use a bed-alarm—a flat strip laid under the sheets that sounds when the person gets out of bed
- place bolts or indoor locks on the bottom or top of doors where the person wouldn't ordinarily look for a lock
- place child safety gates (you might need two levels for height) at top of stairs, porches, and decks
- install door alarm or bell that will sound if the person wanders outside
- make sure the person wears an ID bracelet or carries ID
- register with Alzheimer's Association Safe Return Program
- place a couple of motion-sensors in the bedroom doorway to alert you if the person tries to wander out of the bedroom at night
- ask neighbors to alert you if the person is seen wandering

Hiding or losing things

Dementia produces feelings of acute vulnerability and causes people to become very anxious. They often feel like they are losing something vital and that they have no power over what is happening to them. As a result, some people begin to hide or lose things. Of course, this won't give them back what they lost, but logical thinking diminishes as dementia progresses, and hiding things can be a way of trying to regain some measure of control.

If hiding things makes the person you are caring for feel more secure, don't try to stop them from doing it. Instead, try to manage it in a way that won't be so upsetting to you and your family.

Managing hiding behaviors

Learn which items the person likes to hide and give them duplicates. For example, if your mother hides keys or money, provide her with some unused keys or "play money" to hide.

Avoid clutter and keep the house neat. Clutter often triggers the hiding response.

Place an empty garbage can or wastebasket in plain view for the person to use as a hideaway. This way, you can direct or manage the activity.

Identify favorite hiding places and check them regularly.

Provide calming and safe activities such as folding laundry, dusting, or sanding wood.

Remember: Trying to eliminate or prohibit these kinds of behavior problems will only prove frustrating. The goal is to manage and limit the behavior or, if necessary, distract the person when the behavior becomes unsafe or overly disruptive.

Putting it into practice

What kind of changes can *you* make? Think about the person for whom you are providing care for.

Do they exhibit any of the behaviors described in this chapter?

If so, what are some of the things you can easily do in your home to manage or limit these behaviors?

Are there any other disruptive behaviors that the person you are caring for exhibits that might be managed or limited by some of these techniques?

If so, what are they and what can you do?

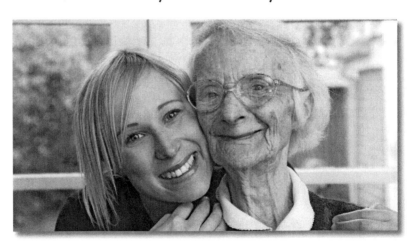

NOTES

Steve,

Thanks so much for all the time you took talking with me today. As I shared with you, you provided me more comprehensive information in our one phone conversation than I have been able to acquire after many telephone conversations with many people at both private organizations (who say they provide social work support information and services) and Missouri state offices.

You provided me tremendous help confirming some of the information I had as well as correcting some of my misunderstandings and helped me put all in an understandable context for Mom's situation.
— Laura

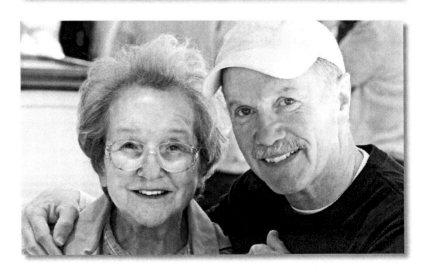

Epilogue

Thousands of families around the world have success-fully used the strategies presented here. These families are just like yours: struggling, grieving over the loss of the person they knew, worrying if they are doing the right thing, but, most important, loving their mother, father, spouse, grandparents, aunt, or uncle. We hope that you tried some (or all) of these strategies. Of course not every strategy or recommendation will always work. So adapt, modify, and make them your own. Remember not to let the past dictate how you address the future. You won't know if it will work unless you try it.

Families that care for their loved ones made this book possible. Families like yours created the strategies and recommendations in this book. The strategies did not evolve in a lab or vacuum, but came from experi-ence caring for someone with dementia, Alzheimer's or memory loss.

People just like you created the ideas and tactics described through trial and error. When you say something that makes your loved one upset or agitated, you know not to say it again. In the future try saying something else and you'll eventually find your right style. Caregivers who learn from their past actions make the strongest caregivers.

We hope this guidebook is a resource for families, provides guidance, and, most important, gives you hope. This book shows how simple ideas, projects, and tasks make a big difference, not only in the life of the person with dementia, but also for the family. Quality of life is essential for the person with memory impairment and for you as a concerned caregiver. We all want what is best for our loved one, but if we don't care for ourselves, then we won't give quality care to our family member.

All caregivers need a break! Finding ways to take time for yourself will help rejuvenate you and keep up your energy and spirits. Remember, small breaks during the day are just as important as a day or weekend respite. If your loved one is doing a task or activity at home for thirty minutes, then you have thirty minutes to do something for yourself. It might not sound like a long time, but it can have an extremely positive effect. When you have more time for yourself, get together with friends, go shopping, take walk in a park, or do whatever gives you pleasure. Remember, the strategies and recommendations in this book are for you. Take advantage of them to extend quality time at home for you and your loved one.

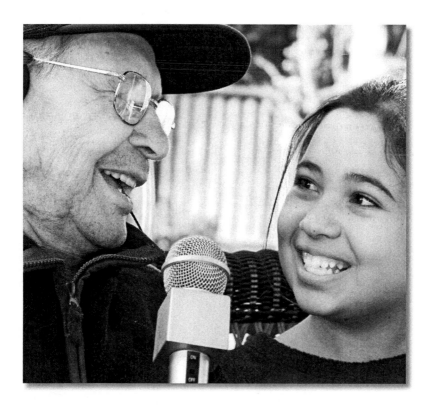

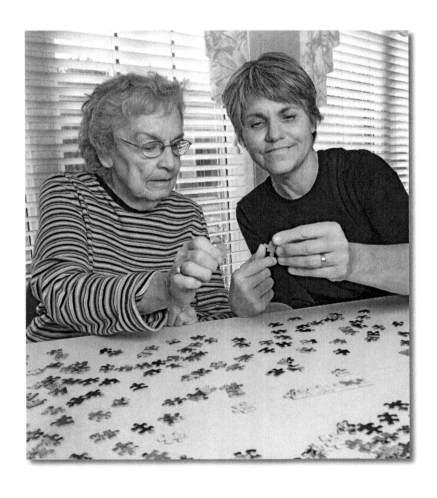

Harriet Rzetelny, LCSW

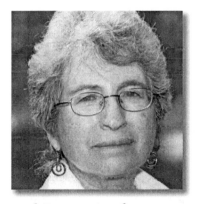

Harriet Rzetelny has practiced, taught and written extensively in the field of aging for over thirty years. After working as a homecare social worker, she was associated with Brookdale Center on Healthy Aging and Longevity for over twenty years. There she developed and taught courses in a wide range of aging subjects including Work with the Frail Elderly, Mental Illness and Aging, Caring for the Caregiver, Reminiscing and Life Review and People in Mid-Life Transitions. Ms. Rzetelny was an Associate Professor at the NYU School of Social Work where she developed and taught the course Work with Aging People and Their Families. In addition, she was the author of training curriculums for NYS Protective Services and the NYS Ombudsman

Program, and also authored the original training curriculum for family caregivers of people with dementia living at home for Memory Care Home Solutions. Aging also figures in her fiction writing: She has recently published a novel featuring a homecare social worker which was based on a series of stories published in *Alfred Hitchcock's Mystery Magazine*. In addition, she maintains a private psychotherapy practice.

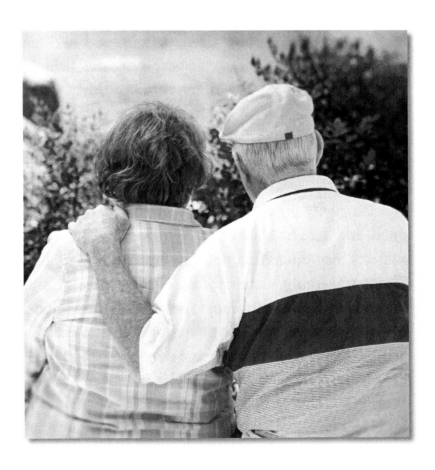

Resources for Family Caregivers

Alzheimer's Association
www.alz.org
1 800-272-3900

Caregiver
www.caregiver.com
1-800-829-2734

Alzheimer's Foundation of America
www.alzfdn.org
1-866-232-8484

Family Caregiver101
www.familycaregiving101.org

Memory Care Home Solutions
www.memorycarehs.org • help@memorycarehs.org
314-645-6247

National Family Caregiver Association
www.thefamilycaregiver.org
1-800-896-3650

National Institute on Health, Senior Health
http://nihseniorhealth.gov
1-888-346-3656

National Institute on Aging Publications
www.nia.nih.gov/HealthInformation/Publications
1-800-222-2225

Health Information from the National Library of Medicine
www.nlm.nih.gov/medlineplus
1-888-346-3656

The Alzheimer's Disease Education and Referral (ADEAR)
www.nia.nih.gov/alzheimers
1-800-438-4380

Memory Care Home Solutions
Ever-increasing demands of caregiving

Memory Care Home Solutions exists to extend and improve quality time at home for families caring for a loved one with memory loss, dementia, or Alzheimer's disease. This mission is achieved through operation of three programs: Customized Caregiver Training and In-Home Consultation, and Education and Outreach.

Customized Caregiver Training is the primary direct service program, which is designed to reduce caregiver stress, promote the functioning ability of the person with dementia and reduce healthcare costs. The program provides in-home assessment and personalized caregiver training that reduces stress for caregivers and allows loved ones with severe memory impairment to remain at home with children and grandchildren, for as long as possible with the best quality of life possible.

The Education and Outreach Program offers free interactive caregiver workshops, presentations and seminars for community, business and civic groups that want to learn more about the options of elder care and our mission.

Our goals

- To reduce family caregiver stress.

- To present the tools, techniques and skills that increase confidence to handle difficult situations.

- To help you prepare and plan for the future.

- To improve quality time at home for you and your loved one.

Contact us today! Memory Care Home Solutions 314-645-6247 • help@memorycarehs.org www.memorycarehs.org

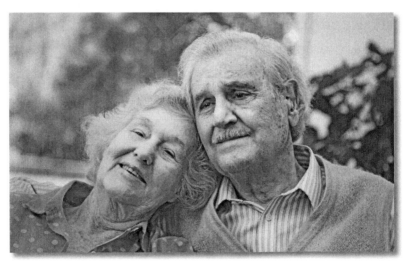

Index

A

B

C

F

facial expressions, 74
failure to recognize the familiar, 45–46
family life, 58
fish tanks, 91
flooring, 89
fluctuating moods, 43–44
4 S's, 77, 81–82
frontal-temporal dementia, 50
functional ability, 55–56, 57, 58–59
functional impairment, 39–40
furniture and wall decorations, 90–91
fuse box metaphor, 49

G

gait and balance, 89
gardening activities, 66–67
gestures, 75

H

habits and preferences, 63
head trauma, 50
hiding behaviors, 104–105
hobbies, 91
home-based caregiving, 19–36
home environment, 32–33
home modification, 85–95

I

ID bracelets, 46, 104

impairments in judgment, 41–42

independence, adult need for, 55–56

K

Koenig Coste, Joanne

    Learning to Speak Alzheimer's, 85

L

language and communications, 47, 81

language limitations, 73–74

Learning to Speak Alzheimer's (Koenig Coste), 85

Lewy body dementia, 50

lighting, 85, 104

long-term memory, 40

M

math calculations, 47

mealtimes, strategies and solutions for, 33–35

Memory Care Home Solutions, 16

memory loss

    dementia and, 39–40

    strategies and solutions for, 41

    modifying activities, 65

    mood swings, 43–44, 64

N

non-verbal communication, 74–76, 91–92

O

orientation to time, place, and person, 46
out-of-pocket costs of care, 16
over-medication, 50–51
over-stimulation, environmental, 48–49

P

Parkinson's disease, 50
pathways, interior, 86, 89–90, 104
physiological changes in the brain, 21–22
pictures and images, 91–92
power of attorney, 48
problems in the home, 23–33

R

reassurance, 79
"recipes," task, 67–68
relaxation techniques, 30
repeated questions, 79–80
reversible conditions, 50
routines, value of, 62

S

T

V

W

NOTES

CPSIA information can be obtained at www.ICGtesting.com
Printed in the USA
LVOW030134041111

253492LV00002B/2/P